A VEGETARIAN LIFESTYLE FOR A MODEL FIGURE

AND

CHEEKBONE SECRETS AND GREAT BEAUTY

by Jan Rose

Dedications

To my friend Robyn, a Nurse, who gave valuable advice about diet, in particular, to senior citizens; and to a beautiful young lady who convinced me by her example that youthful good looks, lovely skin and cheekbones and a model figure can be maintained through the adoption of a vegetarian or vegan way of life.

Consult your Health Practitioner

I am required by law to state that the contents of this booklet are a result of my own personal experience and in no way do I recommend the reader change their diet without first of all consulting their Health Practitioner or Medical General Practitioner.

Preface

When I was in my early twenties living in Melbourne with my husband, I was rushed to hospital one evening with painful abdominal cramps. The prognosis was constipation and so I was treated with the usual helpful drugs for this condition. Soon after this episode I gave up eating meat altogether for several years, and was not hospitalised again for a similar medical condition until I was almost 60 years of age.

During my pregnancy at the age of twenty nine I did supplement my vegetarian produce with fish only and drank copious amounts of soya milk to ensure my diet included adequate protein. I did not gain any excess weight during pregnancy and regained my pre-natal figure soon after the birth of my beautiful baby.

I understand that some people decide that they no longer desire to eat meat and this booklet supplement is written to help educate them on the benefits of converting to a vegetarian or vegan lifestyle, from my own personal experience, rather than make the mistake of omitting to include the valuable sources of plant protein that are required with vegetarian produce.

Table of Contents

Part One

My initial vegetarian diet in the twenties

My diet when I became a vegetarian consisted of vegetables such as carrots, pumpkin, broccoli, sweet potatoes, potatoes, tomatoes, onions, red and green capsicums most days and a grilled slice of vegetarian loaf.   I would also do a pasta dish for my husband and his included beef mince but I would cut up the vegetarian loaf into pieces and add this to my pasta.   Currently I now add a delicious vegetarian mince high in Vitamin B12 and zinc to my spaghetti dish which also includes fresh tomatoes, red capsicum, green capsicum, red chilli, gloves of garlic and red onion.

In all those younger years when I was on the vegetarian diet my weight remained the same, I was always slim, but never too thin.   I was not hospitalised again with the same condition I had prior to adopting my vegetarian lifestyle; nor for any other medical condition; other than when giving birth.

A mistake that some vegetarians may initially make is they do not cut down on full cream dairy products which when consumed in excess, perhaps due to hunger on a vegetarian diet, increases their weight.   Instead of bulking up on products such as potatoes, butter, cheese and other dairy foods because their diet may not include sufficient plant protein, other vitamins and minerals, rather, they should add legumes, tofu, soya beans, wholegrain cereals, nuts and seeds to the fruit and vegetables which form part of their vegetarian lifestyle.

Part Two

A revised vegetarian diet in later years

Tofu was not a food that I found palatable at first, being rather bland, so when I was younger I did not include this in my vegetarian meals until recent years. Firm tofu is best for casserole dishes and this is what I include in delicious stir fry and curry dishes.

I happened to see on a television cooking program about two years ago a handsome young gentleman demonstrating how to make a lentil pie. Ever since I watched that show I have included lentil pies in my vegetarian diet; lentils are a valuable plant food protein source and my version of this recipe is included in a list of vegetarian recipes in this booklet.

Fortunately there appears to be more of a variety of plant protein available at the supermarkets now days than when I was younger and starting on my new eating plan. For instance there is even a Vegie roast loaf, Organic vegetarian mince in a dry texture and a vegetarian casserole mince.

Part Three

Diet deviation and a hospital stay

Several years ago I was admitted to hospital again with abdominal pain. By this time I had included small amounts of chicken and occasionally turkey in my diet. However, as there was left over turkey early one year I had excess amounts and consumed rather more of this than my usual small portion and I believe that this contributed to my diagnosis while in the hospital, with diverticulitis.

The diverticulitis was treated with antibiotics and I was able to go home after about four days. I rarely ever have any flare-ups of this condition and it is now five years ago since I was diagnosed; I have not consumed excess turkey meat since then and have only eaten relatively smaller portions of chicken than I used to.

I deduced from past experience and from reading documentation about meat that in my personal case is definitely true. Meat takes a lot longer to digest than vegetables and it makes sense that my omitting this from my diet has obviously helped my medical condition. The proof is the fact that I have not suffered acutely again from diverticulitis to warrant hospitalisation and it seems to me that my digestive system right from a young age is unable to tolerate meat.

Another food item I have been unable to eat since a child aged seven, is butter. I would gag if I was served bread and butter or any food cooked or fried in butter. At a tender young age I announced I would no longer eat this dairy produce; so parents if your child decides they do not like butter, do not force them to eat it. Follow the example of my intelligent, educated relatives who accept that their children just simply do not want to eat butter at all.

Part Four

Lifetime benefits of my vegetarian diet

Sadly, when I look around at middle-aged and senior people today there are so many who appear to have prematurely aged.   Some are overweight and their skin is wrinkled and their faces puffy; many of them have not spent a lot of time exposed to the sun so it may be true that these are indeed the effects of a poor diet which includes food that I just do not consume at all and certainly not in excess.

I have maintained the same weight for decades and my diet has hardly altered from the age of twenty six when I initially omitted all meat in my diet except for during pregnancy and later years when I added fish and small portions of chicken.   I have not aged prematurely at all and I do enjoy alcohol but limit my intake of this and do not drink every day because I read that alcohol inhibits the body's ability to shed fat.   On those rare occasions throughout my life when I have over indulged on alcohol I have added weight to my figure and have quickly rectified this and reduced my alcohol intake.

My friend Robyn, the Nurse used to say to all her senior patients that if they ate a banana or a few strawberries every day they would still receive all their daily nutrition needs from either of these two fruits.   I guess that some people must find it hard to eat a lot of foods if they have lost their teeth over the years and these were most likely the targeted group to whom Robyn gave this advice.

Vegetarians should eat a variety of fruit, vegetables and plant protein foods to ensure they are getting all the essential vitamins, minerals, iron and amino acids they require daily. I have managed to stay healthy and have subsisted on the following vegetarian recipes for a major portion of my life.

Part Five

Vegetarian Recipes

Breakfast Staple

A half cup of Quick Oats

One cup of soya milk

Sliced banana

Spoonful of organic honey

Sprinkling of cinnamon sugar

Heat the oats and half cup of soya milk, banana and honey for one or two minutes. Add the other half cup of milk and sprinkle the cinnamon sugar on top.

Lentil Pie (makes up four small or one large pie)

One cup of green lentils

One cup of red lentils

Chopped, medium size portion of pumpkin, potato, one medium size red onion, one carrot and a stick of celery.

Cold-pressed olive oil.

Frozen 25% reduced fat puff pastry for vegetarians; this contains only vegetable oils or you can make your own pastry.

Boil the lentils in two separate saucepans on low heat for up to 40 minutes, although red lentils take less time to cook, drain excess liquid.

In a large frying pan add some cold-pressed olive oil and all the chopped up vegetables and cook until light brown, then add the cooked red and green lentils to this mixture.

Line either four small pie containers or a pie plate oven dish with the olive oil and place a layer of puff pastry on the bottom, then add all the cooked vegetarian mixture and another layer of pastry on top.

Cook in a pre-heated oven on 200 Celsius for electric oven or for gas usually at a temperature up to 10-20 Celsius lower for about 8 to 12 minutes until the pastry browns. Serve with salad greens or broccoli.

Tofu or Vegie Roast Stir Fry

Firm tofu or Vegie roast loaf cut into cubes.

Thai Lemon Sauce

Sliced chopped cabbage, red onion, celery, cauliflower, broccoli, snow peas, red capsicum, green capsicum and carrot into stir fry pieces or buy a packet of ready prepared stir fry vegetables.

Sprinkle cold-pressed olive oil into a large frying pan and add all the sliced vegetables and tofu or Vegie roast cubes and lightly cook all together.

Add the Thai lemon sauce and simmer the vegetables and tofu/vegie roast cubes for about 10 to 20 minutes.

Serve with Noodles.

Tofu Curry

Firm tofu cut into cubes

Baby spinach leaves

Carrot cut into rings

Zucchini sliced in rings

Red onion sliced

Pumpkin or sweet potato cut into cubes.

Thai Green Curry Sauce or prepare a curry sauce

Fry the vegetables and tofu in a large pan with cold-pressed olive oil until lightly browned.

Prepare curry sauce by mixing together the following ingredients:

Cornflour

Water

Curry powder

Tablespoon of organic honey.

Add the Thai Green Curry sauce or prepared curry sauce to the vegetable and tofu mixture and simmer for 10 to 15 minutes, only slowly add a small amount of hot water during the simmering stage to the **prepared curry mixture** to ensure it is not too thick.

Serve with Jasmine Rice and uncooked baby spinach leaves on top.

Vegie mince Pasta

Portion of either Spaghetti No 1 or Penne

Bring water in a saucepan on top of the stove to boil then add pasta to cook for up to 10-12 minutes, drain water and pour pasta into a casserole oven dish.

Three fresh tomatoes

A red onion

Half a red capsicum

Half a green capsicum

One Red chilli

Two cloves of fresh garlic.

Half or a full can of the Vegie casserole mince.

Cut up and slice all the vegetables and cook with the vegie mince in cold-pressed olive oil until golden brown in a large frying pan on top of the stove.

Add the vegie mince and vegetables mixture to the cooked pasta in a casserole oven dish and heat in the oven at 180 Celsius electric and lower temperature for gas for up to 8 minutes.

Serve on dinner plates and add a small amount of tomato sauce to the dish if you desire.

Roast vegetables and risotto

Bake potatoes, pumpkin pieces, parsnips, carrots and red onions, in an oven on 200 Celsius electric and a lower temperature for gas for up to 35 minutes, turning the vegetables over once during baking.

Rissoto – Brown rice boiled in a saucepan on top of the stove for 35 minutes. Drain and add the rice into an oven casserole dish with separately steam cooked sweet potato, baby spinach, eggplant, celery and grated cloves of garlic.

Place the casserole dish with the risotto into the oven and roast on 180-200 Celsius for up to fifteen minutes.

Serve the Rissoto with the roast vegetables and steamed broccoli.

Vegetarian Lasagne

Lasagne sheets to cover an oven casserole dish in three layers.

One cup from a packet of dry organic vegetarian mince

Vegetarian cheese grated

Fresh tomatoes

Half each of a red, yellow and green capsicum

One or two cloves of garlic

Fresh Oregano leaves

Fresh parsley

One red onion.

Prepare the cup of dry organic vegetarian mince by boiling in two cups of water on top of a stove and simmering for up to 5 minutes, then stand for ten minutes and afterwards drain the water.

Slice the tomatoes, onion, capsicums and garlic and cook in cold-pressed olive oil in a large frying pan on top of the stove until light brown. Add the prepared vegetarian mince, oregano and parsley to the mixture and stir in a small tub of tomato paste and simmer in the pan for up to fifteen minutes on the stove.

Line a casserole dish with olive oil and a layer of lasagne sheets, then a layer of the vegetarian mixture, and sprinkle grated vegetarian cheese on top, then add another two layers of the lasagne sheets and vegetarian mixture and sprinkle the grated vegetarian cheese on top of each added layer.

Bake in a pre-heated oven 150-160 Celsius for about 30-35 minutes.

Serve with a garden salad.

Desserts

A serving of any of the following fruits: fresh or dried blackberries, blueberries, raspberries, apples, bananas, kiwi, pears, plums, oranges, strawberries, peaches, apricots, papaya or paw paw, nectarines and grapes.

A serving of the following nuts/seeds: almonds, walnuts, cashews, sunflower seeds or pumpkin seeds.

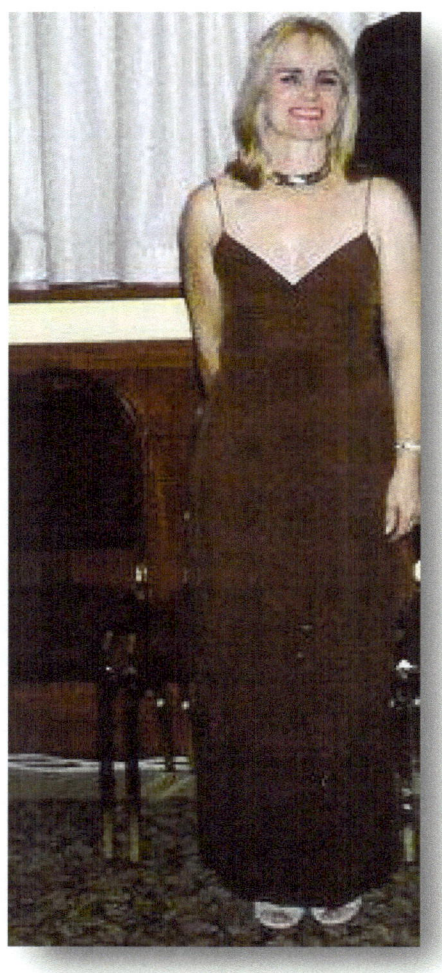

Jan Rose, author of "A Vegetarian Lifestyle for a Model Figure" which is a supplement to her previous booklet "Cheekbone Secrets and Great Beauty" has another title "My Jasmine Rose" which is about her pet dog and also available on Amazon.com. She gained a Major in Commercial Law at the University of South Australia in her Bachelor of Business degree and her interest in a career as a writer was inspired by studies in communication and media at University.

CHEEKBONE SECRETS AND GREAT BEAUTY

by Jan Rose

Dedications

To the heroines and heroes of my youth, in particular the English model Jean Shrimpton and Dennis, the young lawyer I once loved long ago.

TABLE OF CONTENTS

Part 1

Definition of cheekbones and ideal face

Research on beauty and cheekbones reveals that the ideal face according to a census conducted is big wide-set eyes, strong jawline which narrows at the chin, high and or prominent cheekbones, a straight, narrow nose and generous cupid bow shaped lips.   The sixties model Jean Shrimpton was the epitome of great beauty, named the most beautiful woman in the world in her heyday, she had all the perfect facial features that match the criteria of an ideal beautiful face.

Chubby faces, on the other side of the spectrum, do not have the face "cut" that is considered a hallmark of great beauty. For a start the cheekbones are often indefinable on such a face and in Part 5 of this article I list the ways and means to achieve a more desirable facial structure.

Most models have high cheekbones and or prominent or wide cheekbones as they look extremely attractive in photos; the camera highlights the angular structure of the face. This lighting whether it is daylight or special effects lighting, captures high cheekbones and as a result they look stunning.

If you are still young your cheekbones may not have fully developed but as you mature they can become more prominent; there are factors which will influence the definition of this facial trait listed in Part 5. In old age a person with small high cheekbones appears to have a hollow look of sunken cheeks if the face lacks fat in this area.   So although high cheekbones are a highly desirable trait of great beauty in youth, unless they are also wide or prominent cheekbones then their facial structure will not maintain as youthful an appearance in later years.

Part 2

Description of various cheekbones

High, wide-set, prominent or large cheekbones result in a sculptured look and cut to the face giving definition; it is a fact that the majority of people have medium or lower set cheekbones and if also wide-set and large or prominent then they too are very attractive and a great aid to keeping the face more youthful looking into old age. It is the luck of the genes though as high or wide-set, prominent cheekbones are usually hereditary.

My mother inherited wonderful wide-set, prominent cheekbones from her father and my grandfather from his father also.   I inherited my high, wide-set, prominent cheekbones also from my mother, grandfather and great-grandfather; however, the high cheekbones were also in my father's genes.   My daughter has inherited these same cheekbones which will become even more developed as she grows older.

The talented singer Cher has wide-set, prominent cheekbones as well as beautiful eyes.   Overall though, those celebrities whether male or female who possess a face with beautiful features have either high or wide-set, prominent cheekbones, beautiful eyes and generous lips like actors Adam Brody, Jonathan Bennett, Benedict Cumberbatch, James Haven and his sister, Angelina Jolie, Keira Knightley and Charlize Theron.

Part 3

Examining facial features and beauty

First of all a face which is symmetrical is considered the most attractive so it bears witness that the structure of a face which includes the cheekbones and their size would need to be evident to be classed as a great physical beauty asset.

Next in order of features that are the hallmark of a beautiful face according to consensus are wide-set large eyes, preferably deep set. No matter what the colour, although violet eyes like those possessed by the beautiful Elizabeth Taylor are rare and therefore considered perhaps as the most desirable colour, this is not the only characteristic which sets the eyes apart from other features.

Naturally long, dark eyelashes framing the eyes adds to the beauty of the eyes, so even if the colour may be violet or turquoise, if the eyelashes are short or average then this will not highlight the beautiful colour. Brown, grey, green or blue eyes will still look stunning if they are also teamed with lovely long dark eyelashes.

The shape of the eyebrows also adds to the beauty effect, if they are high and arched and the brow is a greater distance from the eyelids.

Lips are next in the line-up of the most favoured facial features a generous upper and lower lip in the shape of a cupids bow is highly regarded. A beautiful set of teeth when smiling and showing none of the gums completes the lips and mouth definition of great beauty, like Whitney Houston, who had exquisite teeth and a stunning smile.

The most attractive nose is a straight, well-formed and narrow nose with a length in keeping with the symmetry of the entire face. A strong jawline, narrow chin and a neck with a large apple are the most coveted, as these particular areas are most prone to aging, which may eventually result in a double chin, sagging jaw and neck in middle or old age. A long neck is considered beautiful if slim and free of lines and with the presence of the prominent apple as this maintains a youthful neck appearance with care, even in the senior years.

Lovely skin and hair are easier to achieve than perhaps some other facial features and if present, then this is an added bonus to beauty. Singer, Barbra Streisand who has an extraordinarily beautiful voice, has lovely skin, blue eyes and cheekbones and looks amazing in her latest film.

Part 4

Celebrities and their best facial features

There are as many gorgeous men with high and or prominent wide-set cheekbones as there are lovely ladies. From a list of some selected celebrities, although there are many who possess outstanding facial attributes, a brief outline is given of their best features as follows:

Jean Shrimpton with her exquisitely big, beautiful wide-set green eyes and long red hair was sought after as a photographic model due to her amazing facial structure; high, wide-set prominent cheekbones, arched eyebrows, generous lips, strong jawline, narrow chin and long neck with a prominent apple.

Angelina Jolie has beautiful wide-set prominent, high cheekbones, her mother Marcheline also had the same lovely features, as well as beautiful wide-set blue eyes, framed by arched eyebrows, a perfect nose and generous lips.

Grace Kelly, who captured the heart of a Prince, was another very beautiful lady with lovely wide-set blue eyes, wide-set prominent cheekbones, a strong jawline, generous lips and a long neck.

Keira Knightly, an English actor has beautiful dark eyes, framed by lovely long black eyelashes and high, wide-set cheekbones; she should with care, age beautifully with her square shaped strong jawline and lovely long neck and prominent apple.

Miranda Kerr, a stunning young model, has beautiful blue eyes, lovely skin and wide-set cheekbones and a perfect jawline and neck.

At the top of my male list is a Japanese actor and musician, Gackt, who has stunning high, wide-set cheekbones and arched eyebrows.

Adam Brody, also an actor has high and prominent wide-set cheekbones, beautiful eyes and generous lips.

Jonathan Bennett, actor, also has stunning high, wide-set cheekbones and generous lips.

Benedict Cumberbatch, another English actor, famous for his modern day, wonderful portrayal as Sherlock Holmes, is also admired for his amazing high, prominent cheekbones.

River Phoenix is added to the list as he had male model facial features with his wide-set prominent cheekbones; incidentally, it is documented that he was a vegetarian.

Cheekbone Secrets and Great Beauty

A major factor which affects the skin throughout life is first and foremost Diet. The detrimental effects of the sun can be a contributing factor if out in the sunshine for extended periods of time, but this is not to say that the sun is to be avoided altogether because sunshine is needed for Vitamin D.

Studies as well as personal experience have revealed to me, and verified by medical documentation that to avoid premature ageing a nutritious diet of fruits, nuts, vegetables, legumes, oats, wholegrain cereals, tea and cold pressed olive oil will slow ageing. In fact the Vegan diet which mainly consists of raw vegetarian products and no dairy is best and is a diet which is even followed by some celebrities.

I am acquainted with a beautiful young lady through family connections who has "cheekbones to die for", beautiful skin and a model figure; her beauty secret is the fact that she is a total Vegan, her diet consists of only raw fruit, nuts, legumes and vegetables and no meat or dairy produce.

Foods that should be avoided are fatty processed meat, full-fat dairy products, butter, sugar-laced pastries, cakes, soft drinks and potatoes as these all contribute to premature ageing and this has also been documented.

I hardly eat any meat at all, in fact only an occasional small serve of chicken or fish and have not consumed lamb, pork, ham, bacon, beef or any other meat for thirty-nine years and no butter since the age of seven, and I am told I look sixteen years younger than my actual age.

I wish to retain visible definition of my high, wide-set cheekbones and so I choose to promote good looks over junk food and anyway, it is documented that eating meat adversely affects the skin causing premature ageing. I agree with this fact because in my experience not eating meat has resulted in a youthful appearance as evidenced by the recent photo taken of me which appears on the last page.

An excellent makeup trick to accentuate the cheekbones even if they are not a prominent feature of your face is to highlight directly under the eye area with a white concealer or blush, next add a pale pink blush under the white, and apply a darker blush in pink or beige under the hollow of the cheek. This is an inexpensive method used to give a prominent cheekbone effect. An expensive option is to have cheekbone implants performed by a plastic surgeon.

Another make-up technique which can be used to give the lips the illusion of a more generous size is to outline upper and lower lips with a lip stain as this lasts for hours, and then apply a light lipstick colour over the lip stain when it is dry.

Sudden fluctuations in weight gain adversely changes the skin and appearance which will mean that it will be harder to regain your earlier youthful looks; the exception is in pregnancy as it is natural for an expectant mother to gain a little extra weight on a recommended nutritious diet.

Walking is recommended as a wonderful gentle form of exercise as exercise is essential for strong bone density, when I was young I used to walk ten kilometres a day to and from home and my place of employment. Also to maintain height I have ever since I was a young girl performed a nightly exercise where I lie down and raise the legs right over the head to gently stretch the spine, keeping the knees straight and stretching the arms towards the feet.

In addition to a nutritious diet, and it is better to only eat when hungry, drink adequate water each day, exercise on a regular basis and limit alcohol intake. It is important to note that beauty is more than just having good bone structure and lovely facial features, it begins on the inside with the right food intake, but also we should strive to be kind, compassionate and humble to promote inner beauty which lasts a lifetime.

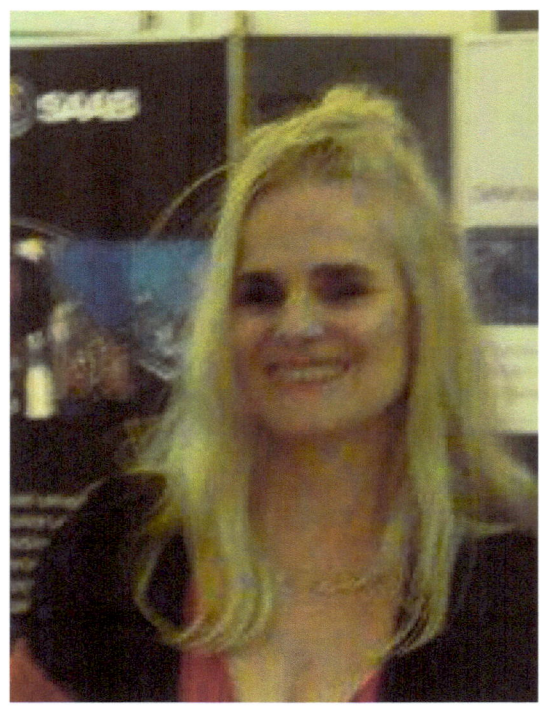

Jan Rose, author of "My Jasmine Rose" available on Amazon.com and a new title "A Journey through Time" soon to be published on Amazon.com in March 2013, gained a Major in Commercial Law at the University of South Australia in her Bachelor of Business degree. Jan credits her interest in a career as a writer was inspired by studies in communication and media at University.

www.ingramcontent.com/pod-product-compliance
Lightning Source LLC
Chambersburg PA
CBHW060824290526
45792CB00005BB/1794